THE ACUPRESSURE FOR WEIGHT LOSS GUIDE

GEORGE ANDERSON

The Author hereby reserves all rights provided by copyright law, including but not limited to the rights to reproduce, distribute, display, and create derivative works of the copyrighted book. Any unauthorized use, reproduction, or distribution of the book or its content without the express written consent of the Author is strictly prohibited and may result in legal action.

This Notice is without prejudice to any additional or more specific terms that may be included in a separate licensing agreement between the Author and a third party.

CHAPTER ONE

INTRODUCTION

Acupressure

Acupressure (Chinese -Tui na), is an alternative medicine technique often used in conjunction with acupuncture or reflexology. It is based on the concept of life energy which flows through "meridians" in the body. In treatment, physical pressure is applied to acupuncture points or ashi trigger points with the aim of clearing blockages in these meridians. Pressure may be applied by hand, by elbow, or with various devices.

Although some medical studies have suggested that acupressure may be effective at helping manage nausea and vomiting, insomnia, low back pain, tension headaches, stomach ache, among other things, such studies have been found to have a high likelihood of bias. There is no reliable evidence for the effectiveness of acupressure.

BACKGROUND OF ACUPRESSURE

Acupoints used in treatment may or may not be in the same area of the body as the targeted symptom. The traditional Chinese medicine (TCM) theory for the selection of such points and their effectiveness is that they work by stimulating the meridian system to bring about relief by rebalancing yin, yang and qi (also spelled "chi").

Many East Asian martial arts also make extensive study and use of acupressure for self-defense and health purposes, (chin na, tui na). The points or combinations of points are said to be used to manipulate or incapacitate an opponent. Also, martial artists regularly massage their own acupressure points in routines to remove supposed blockages from their own meridians, claiming to thereby enhance their circulation and flexibility and keeping the points "soft" or less vulnerable to an attack.

INSTRUMENTS FOR ACUPRESSURE

There are several different instruments for applying nonspecific pressure by rubbing, rolling, or applying pressure on the reflex zones of the body. The acuball is a small ball made of rubber with protuberances that is heatable. It is used to apply pressure and relieve muscle and joint pain. The energy roller is a small cylinder with protuberances. It is held between the hands and rolled back and forth to apply acupressure. The foot roller (also "krupa chakra") is a round, cylindrical roller with protuberances. It is placed on the floor and the foot is rolled back and forth over it. The power mat (also pyramid mat) is a mat with small pyramid-shaped bumps that you walk on. The spine roller is a bumpy roller containing magnets that is rolled up and down the spine. The Teishein is one of the original nine classical acupuncture needles described in the original texts of acupuncture. Even though it is described as an acupuncture needle it did not pierce the skin. It is used to apply rapid percussion pressure to the points being treated.

ACUPRESSURE POINTS AND MASSAGE TREATMENT

Used for thousands of years in China, acupressure applies the same principles as acupuncture to promote relaxation and wellness and to treat disease. Sometimes called pressure acupuncture, Acupressure is often thought of as simply acupuncture without the needles. But what exactly is acupressure and how does it work?

What Is the Theory Behind Acupressure?

Acupressure is just one of a number of Asian bodywork therapies (ABT) with roots in traditional Chinese medicine (TCM). Examples of other Asian bodywork therapies are medical qigong and Tuina. Shiatsu is a Japanese form of acupressure.

Traditional Chinese medical theory describes special acupoints, or acupressure points, that lie along meridians, or channels, in your body. These are the same energy meridians and acupoints as those targeted with acupuncture. It is believed that through these invisible channels flows vital energy or a life force called qi (ch'i). It is also believed that these 12 major meridians connect specific organs or networks of organs, organizing a system of communication throughout your body. The meridians begin at your fingertips, connect to your brain, and then connect to an organ associated with a certain meridian.

According to this theory, when one of these meridians is blocked or out of balance, illness can occur. Acupressure and acupuncture are among the types of TCM that are thought to help restore balance.

How Does Acupressure Work?

Acupressure practitioners use their fingers, palms, elbows or feet, or special devices to apply pressure to acupoints on the body's meridians. Sometimes, acupressure also involves stretching or acupressure massage, as well as other methods.

During an acupressure session, you lie fully clothed on a soft massage table. The practitioner gently presses on acupressure points on your body. A session typically lasts about one hour. You may need several sessions for the best results.

The goal of acupressure or other types of Asian bodywork is to restore health and balance to the body's channels of energy and to regulate opposing forces of yin (negative energy) and yang (positive energy). Some proponents claim acupressure not only treats the energy fields and body but also the mind, emotions, and spirit. Some even believe that therapists can transmit the vital energy (external qi) to another person.

Not all Western practitioners believe that this is possible or even that these meridians exist. Instead, they attribute any results to other factors, such as reduced muscle tension, improved circulation, or stimulation of endorphins, which are natural pain relievers.

WHICH HEALTH PROBLEMS BENEFIT FROM ACUPRESSURE?

Research into the health benefits of acupressure is in its infancy. Many patient reports support its use for a number of health concerns. More well-designed research is needed, though. Here are a few health problems that appear to improve with acupressure:

Nausea. Several studies support the use of wrist acupressure to prevent and treat nausea and vomiting:

• After surgery

• During spinal anesthesia

• After chemotherapy

• From motion sickness

• Related to pregnancy

The PC 6 acupressure point is located in the groove between the two large tendons on the inside of the wrist that start at the base of the palm. There are special wristbands that are sold over the counter. These press on similar pressure points and work for some people.

Cancer. In addition to relieving nausea right after chemotherapy, there are individual reports that acupressure also helps reduce stress, improve energy levels, relieve pain, and lessen other symptoms of cancer or its treatments. More research is needed to confirm these reports.

Pain. Some preliminary evidence suggests that acupressure may help with low back pain, postoperative pain, or headache. Pain from other conditions may benefit, as well. To relieve headache, the LI 4 pressure point is sometimes tried.

Arthritis. Some studies suggest that acupressure releases endorphins and promotes anti-inflammatory effects, helping with certain types of arthritis.

Depression and anxiety. More than one study suggests that fatigue and mood may improve from the use of acupressure. Better designed trials are needed to be sure.

PRECAUTIONS WITH ACUPRESSURE

In general, acupressure is very safe. If you have cancer, arthritis, heart disease, or a chronic condition, be sure to have a discussion with your doctor before trying any therapy that involves moving joints and muscles, such as acupressure. And, make sure your acupressure practitioner is licensed and certified.

Deep tissue work such as acupressure may need to be avoided if any of the following conditions apply:

• The treatment is in the area of a cancerous tumor or if the cancer has spread to bones

• You have rheumatoid arthritis, a spinal injury, or a bone disease that could be made worse by physical manipulation

• You have varicose veins

• You are pregnant (because certain points may induce contractions)

THE BENEFITS AND USES OF ACUPRESSURE

Acupressure is a traditional Chinese medicine (TCM) practice that involves treating blocked energy, or qi, by applying manual pressure to specific points on the body. It is similar to acupuncture, except that it uses fingertip pressure instead of needles.

By improving energy flow, acupressure is said to help with a range of conditions, from motion sickness to headache to muscle pain.

This book looks at acupressure, its uses, and the evidence for its effectiveness. It also discusses safety and technique.

How Does Acupressure Work?

No one is sure exactly how acupressure might work. Some think the pressure may cause the release of endorphins. These are natural pain-relieving chemicals in the body.

Others think the pressure may influence the autonomic nervous system. This is the part of the nervous system that controls involuntary things like your heart, digestion, and breathing.

According to the principles of TCM, invisible pathways of energy called meridians flow within the body. At least 14 meridians are thought to connect the organs with other parts of the body.

Acupressure points lie along those meridians. If qi is blocked at any point on a meridian, it's thought to cause health problems along that pathway.

A practitioner applies pressure to specific acupressure points to restore healthy energy flow. The points they choose depends on your symptoms.

Given how meridians run, pressure points used may be a long way from the site of the symptom. For example, an acupressure point on the foot may be used to relieve a headache.

CHAPTER TWO

How to Massage Your Pressure Points

When you have localized pain, what do you do? You reach for it. Often without conscious thought, your hand goes to the area of discomfort and massages it. Understanding the basics of acupressure could make this mindless self-massage even more beneficial, helping you to relax and even manage chronic pain.

Acupressure has its foundation in traditional Chinese medicine (TCM), where it has been in use for over 2,000 years. It's a method of activating the body's self-healing mechanisms to treat illness and alleviate pain. Like acupuncture, which uses tiny needles, acupressure stimulates the body at certain meridians, or pressure points.

"The Chinese medical model discovered that the human body is crisscrossed by these invisible lines of energy," explains Dr. Steve Moreau, DOM, AP, a licensed acupuncturist and instructor at the Florida College of Integrative Medicine. "TCM theory also holds that each meridian pathway is connected to a specific organ. It's this interconnection of specific points that allows acupressure to work."

Is it effective? The research says yes. One review found acupressure to be effective at reducing pain in nine of ten studies. With a 2,000-year-old track record, this method of pain management has certainly stood the test of time.

ACUPRESSURE FOR WEIGHT LOSS

Acupressure is a practice in traditional Chinese medicine that involves applying manual pressure on specific points on the body. Unlike acupuncture, acupressure practitioners use their fingers, palms, elbow, feet, or other devices instead of needles.

There have been claims that acupressure is effective at helping someone lose weight. While there is little research to confirm this benefit, some studies are showing promising results.

Acupressure is safe for most people who may want to try it as supplementation to a conventional diet and exercise plan.

What Is Acupressure?

A quick recap of what I said earlier in the first part of this book.

Acupressure is part of the ancient practice of traditional Chinese medicine. Practitioners of traditional Chinese medicine believe the human body has 361 acupressure points connected by pathways known as meridians.

An energy flow called qi follows these pathways through the body, which is responsible for overall health. Disruption of the energy flow can cause disease.

By applying acupuncture to certain points, it is thought to improve the flow of qi and therefore health.

Each pressure point can be found along one of the principal meridians:

• Lung meridian

• Large intestine meridian

• Spleen meridian

• Heart meridian

• Small intestine meridian

• Bladder meridian

• Kidney meridian

• Pericardium meridian

• Stomach meridian

• Gallbladder meridian

• Liver meridian

There are also two other meridians that don't fall under the category of principal meridians. These include the governor vessel meridian and conception vessel meridian.

Each meridian lines a pathway to a different organ system and is thought to affect how healthy that system is depending on the level of energy flow.

Studies have shown that acupressure can help with various ailments including headaches, nausea, mood disorders such as anxiety and depression, and chronic pain.

Can It Help You Lose Weight?

Although acupressure has been proven effective for many ailments, the jury is still out when it comes to weight loss.

Traditional Chinese medicine practitioners believe that gaining weight is caused by an energy imbalance within the body. Since acupressure is designed to restore this balance, it is thought that it can help reduce overall weight in people who are overweight or obese and using other ways to lose weight.

Recent research has found that there may be some truth to these claims. It has been found that acupressure points that influence digestion, metabolism, and stress reduction could all play a vital role in the use of acupressure for weight loss.

One systematic review pulled information from seven studies and found that using pressure points on the ear, known as auricular acupoints, aided in the overall reduction of weight over a 12-week period.

4 PRESSURE POINTS FOR WEIGHT LOSS

Acupressure therapy is something that can be done at home. If done properly, it could also lead to health benefits and be a cost-effective and viable supplemental treatment option for those already working toward losing weight.

There are four pressure points, other than the auricular acupoint, that could aid in weight loss. This is, however, an evolving area of study, and many of the benefits are still being investigated.

Tips for Proper Technique

For the therapy to be effective, the proper technique will need to be applied. It's important to find the pressure point and press down until there is resistance without pain. While pressing down, make a circular motion with your thumb using even pressure throughout.

San Yin Jiao (Three Yin Intersection)

The SP6 pressure point can be found on the spleen meridian. It is thought that it has a great effect on the organs in the lower abdomen as well as the parasympathetic nervous system, the system that controls all bodily functions while it is at rest.

The point is located on the inner ankles, about three inches above the ankle bone. Apply firm pressure to the point using one or two fingers, and massage in a circular motion for two to three minutes. For the best results, do the same thing on both the right and left sides.

Zu San Li (Leg Three Mile)

This point is named so because stimulating it would allow farmers to walk an extra three miles. It is located on the front of the leg below the knee. It is found on the stomach meridian.

This could help aid in weight loss by improving digestion. To massage this point, apply firm pressure and massage in a small circular motion for two to three minutes, repeating on both sides.

Tian Shu (Celestial Pivot)

This pressure point can also be found along the stomach meridian. It is located midway between the outer border of the abdominal muscle and the umbilicus line. It is thought to help with gastrointestinal issues such as constipation, diarrhea, and dysentery. It can aid in weight loss by helping regulate the intestines.

Find the point on your abdomen and apply a firm level of pressure. Massage the point in a small and circular motion for two to three minutes, repeating on both sides.

Zhong Wan (Central Stomach)

This point is located not on one of the 12 main meridians, but on the conception vessel meridian. It is thought that this pressure point aids in digestion by influencing the organs in the upper abdomen.

To activate this pressure point, apply firm pressure and massage in a circular motion for up to three minutes.

WHO SHOULDN'T USE ACUPRESSURE?

Although acupressure is considered safe, it should not be used as a first-line treatment for any condition, nor should it be used by everyone. If you are pregnant, you should take caution because certain points can stimulate uterine contractions and may even induce labor. Those with chronic health conditions that involve joint or muscle issues should avoid acupressure prior to speaking with their healthcare provider.

5 ACUPRESSURE POINTS FOR WEIGHT LOSS

Traditional Chinese medicine is widely known for being one of the most practiced holistic health approaches in the world. In the United States, aspects of traditional medicine, such as massage therapy and yoga, are a part of mainstream health and wellness culture.

While many people still use traditional approaches to weight loss, others incorporate holistic practices like acupressure into their weight loss journey.

In this book we'll explore whether acupressure is beneficial for weight loss and how to incorporate acupressure into your weight loss journey.

Acupressure points and weight loss

Acupressure, like acupuncture, is a type of complementary medicine that has long been a part of traditional Chinese medicine practice.

While acupuncture uses needles to stimulate the various pressure points around the body, acupressure is done by stimulating these points through massage therapy.

Acupressure is believed to be effective in reducing stress, boosting digestion, and improving metabolism, all of which play a role in weight management.

Some pressure points are even thought to influence appetite and blood sugar levels, which makes acupressure a potential complement to traditional weight loss approaches, such as diet and exercise.

The meridian energy pathway

In traditional Chinese medicine, each acupressure point on the body exists on an energy pathway called a "meridian." These meridians are named according to the various organs in the body.

Each acupressure point along a meridian is named using the letters corresponding to that meridian, followed by the location of the point on the pathway. These acupressure points also have corresponding traditional names.

Below, you will find some of the acupressure points that are believed to influence digestion, metabolism, and other factors related to weight loss.

1. Zusanli (ST36)

Located along the stomach meridian, zusanli is believed to influence the organs of the upper abdomen, the parasympathetic nervous system (which controls digestion), and the overall energy of the body.

This point is located below the kneecap, roughly 3 inches below and 1 inch away from the center of the body.

To massage this point:

1. Place two fingers on one of the zusanli points.

2. Apply gentle but firm pressure to the point with both fingers.

3. Use a circular motion to massage the point for 2 to 3 minutes.

4. Repeat on the other side.

Share on Pinterest

2. Sanyinjiao (SP6)

Located along the spleen meridian, sanyinjiao is thought to influence the organs of the lower abdomen and the parasympathetic nervous system.

This point is located roughly 3 inches above the inner ankle bone.

To massage this point:

1. Place one to two fingers on one of the sanyinjiao points.

2. Apply gentle but firm pressure to the point with the finger(s).

3. Use a circular motion to massage the point for 2 to 3 minutes.

4. Repeat on the other side.

Share on Pinterest

3. Zhongwan (CV12)

This point is along the conception vessel meridian. Zhongwan is believed to influence the organs of the upper abdomen, as well as those related to digestion, such as the stomach and intestines.

This point is located roughly four inches above the navel.

To massage this point:

1. Place two fingers on the zhongwan point.

2. Apply gentle but firm pressure to the point with both fingers. Be careful to not apply too much pressure to this sensitive area.

3. Use a circular motion to massage the point for 2 to 3 minutes.

Share on Pinterest

4. Renzhong (GV26)

Located along the governing meridian, renzhong is thought to have an influence on weight, especially obesity.

This point is located on the philtrum, less than 1 inch below where the nostrils meet.

To massage this point:

1. Place one finger on the renzhong point.

2. Apply gentle but firm pressure to the point with the finger.

3. Use a circular motion to massage the point for 2 to 3 minutes.

Share on Pinterest

5. Xuehai (SP10)

Located along the spleen meridian, xuehai is believed to have an impact on blood sugar levels, particularly in the context of diabetes.

This point is located above the kneecap, roughly two inches away from the center of the body at the bottom portion of the thigh muscle.

To massage this point:

1. Place two fingers on the xuehai point.

2. Apply gentle but firm pressure to the point with both fingers.

3. Use a circular motion to massage the point for 2 to 3 minutes.

4. Repeat on the other side.

ARE ACUPRESSURE POINTS EFFECTIVE IN WEIGHT LOSS?

The research on acupressure and weight loss is limited. However, the current literature suggests that acupressure may be effective in aiding weight loss for individuals with obesity.

In a small systematic review from 2019, seven studies were analyzed to determine the potential impact of auricular acupressure on weight loss outcomes.

Auricular acupressure is a specific type of acupressure that stimulates the pressure points of the ear. The studies included in the analysis compared the use of acupressure alone (or with other interventions) with other experimental treatments or no treatment.

The authors found that auricular acupressure was effective in reducing both overall body weight (BW) and body mass index (BMI) in study participants.

These results remained consistent whether the acupressure was administered alone or with diet and exercise. They also found that a longer acupressure treatment period was associated with a larger impact on reducing BW and BMI.

What about acupuncture for weight loss?

Like acupressure research, the literature on using acupuncture as a weight loss tool is limited. Still, similar results have suggested that acupuncture may be effective for aiding in weight loss.

In a larger systematic review from 2018, the authors included 21 studies for analysis, with a total of 1,389 study participants.

The studies in this analysis compared the use of acupuncture alone with other interventions, such as medications, diet, exercise, or placebo. Researchers investigated classical acupuncture, along with other variations, such as laser acupuncture and auricular acupressure.

The authors found mixed results among the studies, with some studies demonstrating more effective weight loss from acupuncture and others demonstrating no discernible difference between interventions.

However, the research suggests that acupuncture may have some effect on appetite and the metabolism of hunger-related hormones.

Still, further research is needed on the use of both acupressure and acupuncture as a weight loss intervention.

WHEN TO SEE A DOCTOR

When you're on a weight loss journey, it can be helpful to have a handful of different tools and options at your disposal, such as:

• Dietary interventions. Fad diets can do more harm than good. A licensed nutritionist can help you explore dietary options that will help you stay physically and mentally healthy during your weight loss journey.

• Lifestyle interventions. Keeping active isn't important just for weight loss. Exercise and other physical activities help keep both our bodies and minds strong. Consider exploring different physical activities until you find the ones you really enjoy.

• Holistic interventions. Holistic health approaches can be used in conjunction with western approaches when it comes to weight loss. While more research is still needed on the effectiveness of acupressure, it's something to consider trying.

There's no one-size-fits all approach to healthy weight loss, so it can be helpful to work with a doctor or other healthcare professional to find what works for you.

HERE ARE 4 PRESSURE POINTS TO BOOST YOUR METABOLISM AND LOSE WEIGHT:

1.Upper lip

Apply gentle pressure on the space between your upper lip and nose (philtrum). Make sure to apply moderate pressure right in the centre of the philtrum. This pressure point is known as the shuigou spot.

You can also massage this spot in a circular motion for 2-3 minutes every day to stimulate metabolism.

2. Inner elbow

Bend your arm slightly to locate this point on the inner elbow. This pressure point is located an inch below from the crease of your elbow joint, towards your inner elbow. Press this point daily for 2-3 minutes with your thumb. It helps in stimulating the intestinal function

3. Ear point

To locate this point, simply place your finger where your jaw starts from. Move your jaw up and down and put your finger on the pressure point with the most movement. Press this point with your forefinger for 1-2 minutes daily.

Pressing this point which is located just beneath your earlobe helps in controlling appetite

4. Thumb point

Locate the pressure point on the bottom part of your thumb and apply pressure. It will stimulate the thyroid gland and increase your metabolism. Apply pressure on the point for around two minutes daily.

10 EFFECTIVE WAYS MASSAGE FOR WEIGHT LOSS CAN GET YOU SLIM FASTER

How Massage For Weight Loss Works?

A massage for weight loss can be an excellent way to help you deal with weight loss. Massage heals your body in a thousand ways. The research is still going on on the therapeutic effects of massage for weight loss. Massage also helps you to get rid of excess fat, reduce cellulite, and improve digestion. It is an effective way for obese persons to reduce their weight.

Massage Improves Blood Circulation

Poor blood flow results in the accumulation of waste metabolites in the body that is associated with weight gain.

Massage for weight loss is known to improve blood circulation. There were a total of 28 participants that received a ten-minute massage on the calf area. There was an increase in temperature, which suggested improved blood flow. It can be because of the pressure applied to some areas that move blood through the congested areas.

An increased blood flow carries more oxygen and nutrients to body organs and removes all the toxic metabolites from the body through the kidney as urine. In this way, the increased removal of waste products prevents their accumulation in the body, thus decreasing the chance of weight gain.

Massage Improves Muscle Tone

Many exercises help lower your weight, but sore muscles decrease your performance during exercise. Massage relieves sore muscles; it allows you to perform better during exercise and burn more calories, enhancing your weight loss.

It manipulates your tissues. It improves muscle tone mainly by improving oxygen supply to oxygen through increased blood flow. It also helps tight muscles to loosen, thus decreasing the soreness of muscles.

Combined massage therapy and transcutaneous electrical nerve stimulation were given to 20 healthy subjects. The results verified massage effectiveness in improving muscle tone.

Improves Cellulite Appearance

A massage is also known to improve the appearance of cellulite by stretching skin. Cellulite is a condition where lumpy flesh develops on thighs and buttocks. It is subcutaneous fat. Cellulitis results when you eat food with high fats. It gets deposited in fat cells and expands them, which results in weight gain.

If massage is applied to cellulite targeted areas, it breaks down fat and reduces its appearance that lowers your weight, and makes you look slimmer.

Massage Relieve Stress

Several kinds of research show that increased levels of stress are associated with weight gain. It may be due to an increase in appetite or emotional reactions.

Massage for weight loss helps you manage an increased weight that is associated with high-stress levels. A massage is well known for promoting relaxation. It does that in several ways. It produces dopamine and serotonin in the body, which produces feelings of happiness. It also decreases cortisol levels that are produced in response to stress.

Massage Increases Metabolism

A slow metabolism burns only a few calories, which means more fat gets stored in your body resulting in weight gain. On the other hand, increased metabolism means increased energy consumption by your body, helping you burn some extra calories. Massage improves blood circulation. Increased blood flow results in an increased exchange of materials (nutrients) and oxygens between blood cells and body tissues, thus increasing metabolism.

It allows muscles to burn more calories. By having a massage, you can eat your favorite food without being worried about gaining weight.

Massage Removes Toxins From Your Body

The building up of toxins due to poor circulation is associated with weight gain. Toxins may affect hormones like insulin and cortisol that are involved in metabolism. They can also damage your body's ability to burn fat by damaging mitochondrial enzymes, thus increasing the body's weight.

They can change the circadian rhythm and increase the workload of the liver. All of these factors lead to weight gain.

Massage improves blood circulation with the use of effleurage and petrissage movements, which help reduce the level of toxins from your body. A reduced level of toxins results in a lower weight of the body.

Increases Range of Flexibility

Restrictive movements and lesser flexibility result in decreased performance during exercise, restricting your calorie consumption and weight loss results. It can be due to many reasons. One of the reasons is muscle tightness. But massage also solves your problem here.

Massages reduce muscle pain and help the body to get rid of waste products. It manipulates body soft tissues and increases body temperature. It reduces swelling and helps break adhesion. It stretches body tissues and relieves tension, thus increasing range of motion and flexibility.

Increased flexibility of muscles allows you to do better exercise, which is associated with weight reduction.

Massage Improves Digestion

Digestion of food is the most crucial in maintaining weight. Poor digestion does not properly break down your food and results in the deposition of not properly digested food components in the body, which can cause weight gain. Poor food digestion can also be due to increased levels of stress. Massage decreases sympathetic stimulation and enhances parasympathetic stimulation, which promotes rest and digest condition.

Furthermore, massage over the abdomen increases blood circulation to the stomach, which releases acid that promotes the breakdown of food. Massage also stimulates peristalsis, which pushes the food downward in the body towards the intestine.

Massage Reduce Cortisol Levels

Cortisol is usually produced in the body during stress. But its overproduction can affect the body negatively. It increases appetite, which leads to overeating. It is associated with fat deposition in the abdomen area. Both increased appetite and fat deposition are associated with weight gain.

Massage is an effective way to reduce the fat around your belly. It decreases cortisol levels.

CHAPTER THREE

DIFFERENT MASSAGES FOR WEIGHT LOSS

Swedish Massage For Weight Loss

Swedish massage uses long kneading strokes or tapping on the top layer of muscle. Your massage therapist may focus on particular areas of concern. You can also expect to have a full body massage.

Swedish massage may loosen up your tight muscles. It stimulates your nerve endings and improves blood flow. It also improves your lymph drainage. All these mechanisms collectively enhance your weight loss.

Manual Lymphatic Drainage Massage

Lymph fluid is a part of the lymphatic system that helps the body to eliminate toxic materials in the body. If you have lymphedema due to any problem, you can go for a manual lymphatic drainage massage. It helps lymph in your body to move and remove toxic and metabolic wastes by using light and rhythmic movements.

A regular lymphatic massage keeps your lymphatic system healthy, which is associated with a high metabolic rate. An increased metabolic rate means high-fat burn per minute.

Abdominal Massage For Weight Loss

Many studies suggest abdominal massage for weight loss is effective. It treats constipation, bloating, and diarrhea. It helps treat constipation by relaxing smooth muscles. It improves digestive function.

Vacuum Massage For Weight Loss

Vacuum massage is a way to reduce cellulite. It is done by using a mechanical device that is supposed to lift the suction of the skin. The suction makes the skin fold and increases blood flow to the surface of the skin. The process also enhances lymphatic drainage and removes toxic materials from the body. It smooths irregular skin surfaces, stimulates collagen and elastin production. It boosts the immune system and allows deep tissues to relax.

The massage is based on the Chinese traditional medicine system. The massage session lasts 45 minutes.

Udvarthanam, An Ayurvedic Massage

It is a popular ayurvedic massage for weight loss. This massage breaks down fat in our body. The massage is also called scrub and trim. As the name suggests, it uses herbal powder; it is a deep tissue massage. It improves blood circulation, strengthens muscles, and combat body stiffness.

There are mainly two types of udvarthanam massage.

• Ruksha: This kind of massage uses only dry herbal powder and reduces fat under the skin and cellulite.

• Snigadh: This kind of massage is done using dry powders and oils. It is suitable for people with sensitive skin.

Aromatherapy Massage For Weight Loss

Research published shows that one hour of aromatherapy with some oils reduces abdominal weight and waist circumference.

As the name suggests, aromatherapy is a kind of massage that involves rubbing essential oils onto the skin. Oils for aromatherapy are mostly obtained from extracts of flowers, leaves, fruits, seeds, and barks.

Aromatherapy massage reduces stress and anxiety. It also improves sleep and muscle movement. It is associated with reduced appetite. It boosts immunity, treats headaches and migraines.

SUMMARY

Acupressure is a type of traditional Chinese medicine that's believed to have many positive health benefits, including aiding in weight loss.

While the research on acupressure for weight loss is scarce, the current literature suggests that both acupressure and acupuncture may be effective weight loss interventions.

Before you dive into using acupressure for weight loss, reach out to a healthcare professional on how you can best incorporate this practice into your journey.

Since there are a lot of pressure points which help in weight loss, try all the points until you find the one you are most comfortable with. While there is no known side-effect of acupressure, you must stop doing it if you are not comfortable with the results.

Remember that acupressure is just a complementary therapy for weight loss and you cannot use it as a substitute for working out and clean eating.

Acupressure is a safe practice that has been used for thousands of years for a variety of ailments. Some recent research has shown that it could also potentially be a effective weight loss aid.

If you are very overweight or obese, you should always consult with your healthcare provider prior to starting any new treatment or therapy, including acupressure. They can let you know whether it's safe for you to use acupressure.

It's important to remember that acupressure should be used as an additional way to help with weight loss and should not be your only strategy to lose weight. A successful weight loss plan always includes a healthy diet and regular exercise.